Look Who's Talking
A Guide to Esophageal Speech

~Jack Henslee

Preface

Look Who's Talking was first published in 1992 and for several years was issued to incoming students at the annual "International Association of Laryngectomees Voice Institute." After several years of success and two printings interest declined as the tracheoesophageal puncture method of speech rapidly gained in popularity and volume printing became financially unfeasible.

With the advent of electronic publishing it once again became possible to make this manual available to the small audience of laryngectomees and speech pathologists trying to obtain or teach esophageal speech.
Some minor changes have been made to reflect current thinking and technology, but for the most part this is still the original.

Jack Henslee
2014

The Sounds of Silence
~ Jack Henslee

An ominous cancer raged within the darkness.
Yesterday's sun that caressed and nurtured life
Was but a distant memory lost.
A storm of despair and fear was conceived in fury
As I prepared for the sounds of silence.

The lightning struck as a surgeon's knife.
Destruction was swift and final
To flesh, and dreams of future life.
Thoughts of rising from the pain and fear
Were thunderous sounds of silence.

The terror of death subsided within the eye,
Replaced with self pity and surrender.
An exodus of pride and dreams
Bred malignant tumors of apathy in the mind,
As I accepted the sounds of silence.

It was easy to forsake confidence
Then slip into the shadows of the tempest.
Yesterday's dreams became thoughts of failure
As lost ambition poisoned the mind and soul.
Despair and pain were born from the sounds of silence.

The light struggled through slowly at first,
Just enough to reflect some silver in the clouds.
As rays of hope melted the indifference
Particles of esteem and self worth fused together,
Like a laser attacking the sounds of silence.

A vibrant rainbow embraced the passing storm.
Powered by the music of children's laughter,
Supported by love, faith and encouragement.
It lights the gateway to the impossible dream,
A challenge is issued to the sounds of silence.

Dawn brings a new day, a new life,
Like ivory swans rising on thermals of promise.
Successes path will be lined with failure's thorns,
But roses will blossom every few miles.
Victory is certain over the sounds of silence.

Today is a kaleidoscope of love and life,
Filled with opportunity and rewards of endless vision.
I no longer cringe and hide from the pain of silence,
The quest for speech once lost, is fulfilled.
Only a distant echo remains of the sounds of silence....

INTRODUCTION

I was first diagnosed as having cancer of the larynx in 1979 at the uncommonly young age of 34. At that time I had one vocal cord removed, but due to some reconstructive surgery I did not have to undergo a total laryngectomy.

After about two weeks I was able to speak with a very husky type voice at a very low volume. Approximately two months later I was able to speak at a normal level but I could not raise my voice very loud. I remained at this level for nine years, and at that time I had a reoccurrence of the cancer.

This time I was not as lucky. The cancer was too advanced for selective surgery so I had to have a total laryngectomy with a modified radical neck dissection. During the time that I was in the hospital I decided that I was going to try to learn esophageal speech. This decision was influenced by the various pamphlets provided by the American Cancer Society, the encouragement given by my doctor, the speech pathologists at the University of California Davis Medical Center, and most of all, my wife.

I started taking speech therapy at the U.C. Davis Medical Center about six weeks after my surgery. I only had about five 30 minute sessions during a three month period because of the distance I had to drive. During this time I could only speak single syllable words via the consonant injection method or by swallowing air directly into my stomach.

Four months after my surgery I was accepted into the speech clinic program at the University of the Pacific in Stockton, Ca. Because of the close proximity to my home I was now able to take therapy twice a week and for one hour at a time. After two weeks I learned how to properly inject air, and from then on my progress was very rapid.

During my quest to acquire my new voice I had the benefit of a professional speech pathologist, several well respected books written for the benefit of laryngectomees, a very good instructional tape on esophageal speech, and the encouragement, enthusiasm and dedication of several UOP student clinicians. However, even though I was able to learn esophageal speech , I feel that it took much longer than it could have because of the difficulty I had in learning how to properly inject air and control it.

There is no question that the methods and books provided to me were successful. Much of what is contained in here has been presented by others in a similar manner. I have merely tried to present some things that I found particularly helpful to me, and hopefully to others.

My primary goal is to provide a therapy concept that will benefit not only the laryngectomee, but the student, teacher, therapist, and anyone else who needs to understand how esophageal speech can be obtained. I will attempt to present a method of learning or teaching esophageal speech that has proven to be successful and is easy to understand. This is a speech instructional guide for laryngectomees and therapists. I have made no attempt to address any of the other problems associated with being a laryngectomee other than those dealing with speech. Other problems faced by new laryngectomees have already been addressed by Edmuund Lauder, Robert Keith, Don Moss, and numerous others. Some of these efforts have addressed the various methods of alaryngeal speech currently available, however, none of them were intended as primary speech guides.

This manual is primarily written in the first person. This is because most of the information provided relates to my personal experiences, successes, and failures. Each laryngectomee learns at a different pace with various degrees of success. We all must learn from each other, as well as from the methods presented in other books, the guidance provided by our therapists, and most of all the experimentation's that we have tried during our practices.

Everything that I say may not fit your particular situation. Some of the things that I say may be contradictory to what some doctors and/or therapists say and teach.   One example of my opinionated views is the fact that I stress that most laryngectomees can learn esophageal speech. However, there are certainly some very valid medical reasons that may prevent some people from learning. These generally result in the inability of the esophagus to produce sound for various reasons. Your doctor, or speech therapist can easily test your ability to produce sound via a nasal insuflation test, and I feel that this should be done before you try to learn.

Esophageal speech requires a lot of hard work, time, and discipline, which in some cases may result in frustration and depression. You should not have to subject yourself to this if you have a physical limitation that is easily determined by prior testing. Find out in advance!

If you do have a limitation it can sometimes be corrected by your doctor through surgery, i.e., a myotomy, and more recently botox injections have been very successful. But, if you don't have a physical limitation the chances are excellent that you can learn if you will work at it.

It may take you longer than someone else, you may require assistance from multiple sources, and you may never become as proficient as you would like to be. I will probably never be satisfied with my voice, and I make public speeches.

I fully understand that all people who are capable of speaking will not achieve speech, and maybe not even voice. In some cases it is the result of insufficient effort or a physical limitation. In other cases it's the result of no speech therapy or maybe even inadequate speech therapy. If this book helps just one person achieve speech, or one therapist learn to teach esophageal speech, I will have accomplished my goal.

CHAPTER 1

SPEECH ALTERNATIVES

ALTERNATIVE 1: NO SPEECH

Even with the advances that have been made with the various electro-larynx devices, voice prosthesis, and esophageal speech therapy, some people still choose not to communicate verbally.

Some of the most common reasons that laryngectomees choose to remain silent are:

a. They are self-conscious about the sound of the mechanical sounding voice produced by an artificial larynx.

b. Some people (primarily women) are uncomfortable with the sound of the voice created via esophageal speech or a voice prosthesis. They don't consider their new voice to be natural and they ignore the fact that silence is what's unnatural.

c. Some people may be unable to properly care for themselves or maintain a prosthesis because of a physical or mental disability, i.e., poor dexterity, or bad health practices.

d. In a few rare cases there may be a physical disability that prevents any type of speech. The best examples are probably the total or partial loss of the tongue or other damage within the pharyngeal cavity.

There are not many options available to those who either choose not to communicate verbally or are unable to do so. Some of those options are:

a. Written communication (although effective its very slow).

b. Sign language (this only works if your audience can understand sign language).

c. Whisper and/or mouth words (this can provide a limited vocabulary).

d. Use gestures (not only limited but also frustrating).

e. Use a combination of the above (you may be able to create a limited language but your audience will probably be limited to a select group of people).

f. There have also been some recent advances in computer technology that allows messages to be displayed on a screen, via a voice synthesizer, or on mobil devices.

Fortunately most people have numerous options available to them, some of which are addressed in the following pages. Remember, speech is natural and easily obtainable by most laryngectomees.

ALTERNATIVE 2: THE ARTIFICIAL LARYNX

The artificial (or electric) larynx has been around for quite a while and provides an easy method of orally communicating in a relatively short time. There are basically two types available: The neck type, and the oral type. Most of these devices are powered by a battery and are commonly referred to as an electro-larynx. There are a couple of other devices that utilize air from the stoma to create noise in the oral cavity, but the electric devices are the most common being used in the USA.

The electro-larynx is a fairly simple concept and is easy to learn. You either place the device against your neck or you place the tube inside your mouth, and you convert the sound that is transmitted into your oral cavity into speech. This is done by exaggerating your mouth movement as you silently mouth the words.

I started using the neck type about thirty days after my surgery. Because of the excessive amount of swelling I had in my neck, it was difficult for me to find a good soft spot for transmitting the sound through my neck. This problem was overcome by placing the electro-larynx against one of my cheeks. Although the quality generally is not as good when you use a cheek instead of the neck, you can still produce a very understandable voice until the swelling goes down.

Don't be discouraged if you can't speak right away. I thought that I would be able to speak immediately and was somewhat depressed when I found out that I couldn't. Like most things that are new to you, it requires a lot of practice to become proficient. After about one week of practice most of the people that were around me a lot could understand me fairly well. After three weeks the majority of the people that I spoke to could understand me. .

I strongly recommend that all laryngectomees start using a artificial larynx of some type as soon as they are physically able unless they expect to start using the TEP soon. Some doctors and therapists may not agree with this because they feel that once a person learns to communicate this way that they may not try other methods such as esophageal speech. I'm sure that this has and will continue to happen, but the importance of establishing some type of oral communication outweighs the risk.

I consider the electro-larynx to be a necessary and very useful aid to assist you while you are learning esophageal speech. My job required that I speak for extended lengths of time on occasion. If I started getting tired or had a problem with an air bubble in my throat, I would switch to my electro-larynx until I could continue with my esophageal speech. I didn't depend on it but I had no problem with using it as a temporary aid.

There are several different brands of electro-larynx available on the market. Some of the more well known ones are the TruTone, Servox, Romet and the Cooper-Rand. Many people have very diverse opinions about which one is the best. Most of the people that I've talked to think that the Servox and TruTone are the best instruments, however, I have found that some people can use any of the instruments equally well. I have also found that instruments with small "Sounding Heads" produce a better neck seal for most new laryngectomees, and the people that use these type seem to learn a little faster than others. However, once they have learned, they can speak with other instruments with little or no problem.

Like most things in life, your ability to speak well is dependent on the amount of effort you are willing to put into it. Every pharyngeal cavity is shaped differently, the texture and shape of each individual neck is different, and each person will produce different sound resonances from the same instrument. This is further complicated by the fact that all instruments of the same brand do not always produce the same quality of sound or pitch.   So, before you run out and buy an electro-larynx that could cost you a lot of money, check with the Cancer Society in your area and see if there is a local laryngectomee club that maintains a loan closet. If there is one available, then you can "try before you buy". Which electro-larynx is really the best? **It's the one that works for you**.

ALTERNATIVE 3: VOICE PROSTHESIS

There are several different voice prosthesis currently being used. I have mixed emotions about the use of a voice prosthesis because I personally feel that you can learn esophageal speech if you are able to speak with a prosthesis. I also get upset when I hear that the procedure, tracheo-esophageal puncture (TEP), is done to patients without their informed consent. By informed consent I mean that all of the options were not properly explained to the patient, and in a lot of cases the patient was simply "told" that he or she was going to receive a TEP (or even worse, that they had received a TEP). Whatever speech option we choose should be just that, our choice. This is a very personal decision and I resent any one that thinks they can make that decision for us. However, since it is a very successful method of oral communication, I will discuss how it works and the pros and cons of using it.

The prosthesis is basically nothing more than a small tube with a valve on one end. A small puncture opening is created between the trachea and the esophagus thus creating a small air passage that the tube is inserted into. The valve on the end prevents food and liquids from entering the trachea, while allowing air to enter the esophagus from the lungs.

The valve is worn at all times to prevent the opening from closing, and to prevent leakage from the esophagus into the trachea when swallowing. With a little practice the valve is fairly easy to remove and insert. The people that I have spoken to that use a prosthesis state that it must be removed and cleaned anywhere from three times a day, to once every three months. Different people react to it differently and the life of the valve appears to be highly dependent on how often and well it's cleaned, plus the acidity of the user's body and the presence of yeast infection which attacks the valve.

The initial insertion of the valve normally requires a one day stay in the hospital, and the ability to speak can occur at once in some cases. However, some people require a lot of practice before they can speak, and the help of a speech pathologist.

In order to speak you place a finger over the stoma opening. When you exhale this forces the air from your lungs into the esophagus when you try to speak, and vibrates the mucosa of the esophagus walls, thus creating a sound. That sound is converted into speech, similar to the same way that sound and speech are created with the vocal cords. Usually the quality and volume of the TEP voice is equal or better than the average esophageal speaker and the rate of speech is increased.

   Many people choose this alternative because after one or two months of silence they want or need to speak instantly. This decision is usually made for one of the following reasons:

     a. They are not willing to put in the effort required to learn esophageal speech. Although esophageal speech is not particularly difficult to learn it does require a lot of time and hard work. To become efficient you usually must consistently practice for several months. Unfortunately, a lot of laryngectomees are not willing to make that commitment.

     b. In some cases it may be essential that the laryngectomee regain his communication skills as rapidly as possible because of his job, business, or social requirements. This is particularly true for a salesman or self-employed person whose income is directly related to the ability to effectively communicate.

     c. Some laryngectomees feel that they simply cannot learn esophageal speech. They may have tried and failed, or they may not have tried because they read or heard that it was too difficult. If you have been unsuccessful try again. Go to another therapist, buy another book, obtain an instructional tape or video, find an esophageal speaker that will help you, but don't give up.

   The primary advantages of the prosthesis are:

     a. In most cases it allows you to communicate in a relatively short period of time with a good quality voice because its such a simple method. You just block your stoma and speak almost as before.
     b. All that's required on your part is some minor surgery with little or no therapy or practice for most people.

   The primary disadvantages are:

     a. You will be dependent on a device to speak.

     b. The care and maintenance of the device can be a nuisance.

c. Some people may have disabilities that prevent them from properly caring for themselves or maintaining the prosthesis.

d. You will require the use of one hand in order to speak. (Blom-Singer and Atos make a device that allows speech without the use of a hand, but at the time that this was written a lot of people reported difficulty in maintaining a tight air seal and that only about 30% of the people were successful.)

In general though, the prosthesis is a very viable alternative for most people. It's simple, it's easy to learn, and will probably continue to get better. However, as more and more people try it, I frequently hear stories about people that have problems with it. I personally recommend that anyone considering a prosthesis try esophageal speech first. I think you will find that the satisfaction of obtaining your new voice without any artificial assistance is much more rewarding from a personal view point. **Whatever choice you make, just be sure that it's your choice, and not something you were just told to do.**

ALTERNATIVE 4: ESOPHAGEAL SPEECH

I freely admit that I am biased in favor of esophageal speech. Each laryngectomee must make his own decision of which alternative he will choose. The very fact that you have chosen to communicate orally is a giant step in the right direction. I know that esophageal speech was the right choice for me. Is it the right choice for you? As I said before, whatever method you choose is the right choice, as long as you had the opportunity to make an informed decision without a lot of biased pressure from family and various health care professionals.

The pride and satisfaction that I achieved from being able to communicate without any mechanical assistance was beneficial to my recovery. Your mental and psychological well-being is just as important as your physical well-being. Other advantages are that you will not be reliant on other devices to speak, your hands will be free, and…no batteries required. The rest of this book is intended to help you regain your self-confidence and make you feel good about yourself through the power of natural speech.

Most of you can achieve esophageal speech if you are willing to make "the effort."

CHAPTER 2

WHAT IS ESOPHAGEAL SPEECH ?

Esophageal speech is the act of orally communicating by creating sound in the esophagus. This is done by injecting or inhaling air into the esophagus and expelling the air to vibrate the walls of the esophagus to produce sound. A simplified description would be converting a belch sound into speech.

Contrary to what a lot of people think, esophageal speech is not difficult. It does require a lot of dedication and sometimes monotonous work, and at times the progress may seem very slow and be difficult to see (at least from the perspective of the person learning to speak).

At times you may have a lot of frustration and feel like quitting. You will reach certain levels and not seem to progress any further. On some days you may not even be able to say words or phrases that were easily spoken yesterday; but don't give up! Because once you have trained your body to inject and control air in the esophagus, the act of speaking is fairly easy. I like to compare it to training for a marathon race.

You start out at short distances and one of your first thoughts is " Why am I doing this? " You tire easily. You tell yourself that you have better things to do and your goal seems unattainable at this time. But you keep on going......

As you get stronger you start to increase your distance. You have developed some confidence in your decision and in your ability to reach your goal. Your future progress is limited only by your desire to succeed and your self discipline.

When you finally succeed it's because you conditioned your body and learned how to control and pace yourself. By the time you are half way through your speech exercises you will realize that you speak almost exactly the same as before the surgery. The process of learning esophageal speech is to exercise, train, and condition your body to inject or inhale air into the esophagus and control it. That's why I refer to the therapy sessions as exercises instead of lessons.

Esophageal speech does not require any special skills or talent. Intelligence is not a significant factor. If you could speak before, you can learn to speak again. In order to train your body to speak again you only need the following things:

1. Motivation: The motivation to speak in as natural a voice as possible is probably the most critical requirement for learning esophageal speech. If you do not have the motivation and desire to put in the many hours of practice that are required to learn, then esophageal speech is not a good choice for you. The choice is yours. You and you alone are responsible for the quality of your life. If your choice is an electro-larynx or a voice prosthesis then your level of proficiency will be the result of your attitude and motivation to be successful. The same thing applies if your choice is esophageal speech; Proficiency = attitude and motivation.

It is difficult for me to express exactly what motivated me. Esophageal speech seemed to be a much more natural way of speaking than the other methods. It is not necessarily a better way of speaking, but it seemed better for me, and the challenge was too hard to pass up.

2. Self discipline: This is a very important aspect in esophageal speech training. You must establish a set of obtainable goals and commit yourself to them. You need to schedule a specific amount of practice time at specific times and adhere to that schedule. You must learn to control your anger, frustration, and depression. You can't speak when you are tense or emotional. You must never be satisfied with poor speech production. Repeat words over and over that are not understandable.

The biggest single cause for failure is that people won't practice on their own. I have heard all of the excuses over and over again: I was sick (more time to practice), I had company (so what), I was out of town, and on, and on... Some people never practice unless it's with a therapist, others start out with a lot of dedication but they give up if the progress is slow, or, they have some early success and think that they don't have to work as hard anymore. Without discipline you will fail!!

3. Hard work: How much time and effort are enough? That is very difficult to answer because each individual progresses at a different rate. I feel that anything less than two hours a day is inadequate. During the first couple of weeks you should practice for fifteen to twenty minutes at a time five or six times

a day. As you get stronger increase your time for each session, with fewer sessions each day.

In the beginning I would speak for about fifteen minutes into a tape recorder and then play it back while I rested. During that time I would analyze the work that I had done and make notes of what was good or bad.   Once I was able to speak a few words I increased the length of my sessions to 1 1/2 or 2 hours at a time (half of the time was spent listening) for a total of about thirty hours a week. After I returned to work I dropped down to about twenty hours a week and I maintained that schedule until I could speak at an average rate of about 95 words per minute and an attainable rate of about 120 words per minute.

When I began writing this manual it had been nine months since my laryngectomy. Even though I was an accomplished esophageal speaker I was still practicing at least five hours a week, and I will continue to practice until I'm satisfied that all my goals have been achieved. How hard you work, and how long it will take depends on what your goals are.

C H A P T E R 3

FACTS AND TRIVIA

Before I explain how to speak I would like to present a list of certain facts, procedures, and just general information that will be useful or at least interesting:

1. Do not try speech until normal mechanical swallowing has returned or the Doctor says that it's OK to begin working with esophageal speech.

2. You probably still have all of the physical requirements to produce sound and shape it into speech. The primary difference is that you must now obtain the air necessary for sound production in a different manner.

3. If you normally wear a hearing aid or dentures do not practice without them. It is difficult to learn if you can't hear yourself, and proper pronunciation is hard to do with missing teeth.

4. Pulmonary air (air from the lungs) is of no benefit in producing sound for speech. At first try to disassociate your breathing from your speaking. In time you will learn to co-ordinate your air injections, speech, and breathing into one synchronized action.

5. Your chest, shoulders, and neck must be relaxed with little or no tension in order to speak. The more relaxed you are the less effort is required to speak, and a better quality of voice is obtained. When you start to feel tense and your voice starts to sound strained try doing the following: Slow down, stretch, stand up / sit down, take some slow deep breaths, walk, swallow, sigh, etc.

6. Watch for stoma blast or clunking.

    a. Stoma blast is the sound of air being forced through the stoma when you try to speak. Try to reduce the pressure. **Speak softly!!!**

    b. Clunking is the sound that's created when you take a big air injection and trap it. It may be beneficial to deliberately produce this sound in the beginning because it's a good indication that a correct air injection has occurred.

But once you have learned to properly inject air on demand you should try to learn to suppress this sound.

7. The p, t, and k, as sounds are the easiest to make and may facilitate air intake.

8. A description of a vowel: The letters a, e, i, o, u and y are considered the "hard" or "long" vowels (there are other "short" or "soft" vowel sounds in our language). The tongue position defines the sound. There is no obstruction of the air stream from the teeth or lips to influence the sound.

9. A description of a consonant: Any sound other than a vowel. A complete or partial obstruction of the air stream by the teeth, lips and tongue defines the sound.

10. How to make some common sounds:

a. The (p) sound: The lips are closed until the air is released with a slight explosion.

b. The (t) sound: The tongue tip is placed against the upper gums until air is released with a slight explosion.

c. The (k) sound: The back of the tongue rests against the roof of the mouth until the air is released with a slight explosion.

d. The (s) sound: Air escapes through the upper and lower teeth while the tongue is slightly raised.

11. Good esophageal speakers can talk at a rate of 85 to 120 words per minute. The average is 85-100 per minute.

12. The average for non-laryngectomees is 165 words per minute with a range of 140 to 185.

13. Most esophageal speakers speak at a lower decibel level than they did before surgery.

14. The number of syllables per air injection varies among different speakers, but 9 to 15 is a good goal, and 20 to 25 are possible.

15. A common problem for esophageal speakers is the time delay between the initial air injection and the production of sound. If you have this problem try to speak your first word while exhaling.

16. Hiccups may be a problem at first. This usually occurs if you are injecting the air into your stomach (swallowing air) instead of trapping it in the esophagus. It is inevitable that some air will get into the stomach but you should be able to minimize the amount and prevent the hiccups.

17. Air bubbles were, and still are, my biggest problem. Air bubbles are created when saliva and mucus are trying to fill the same space in your throat as the air you injected into your esophagus. The result is a gurgling sound when you speak. I wish I could tell you how to overcome and/or control this problem, but I have not found the ultimate solution yet. The following are some actions that sometime work for me:

    a. Take a drink of water (carbonated beverages help create air bubbles).

    b. Lightly massage your throat.

    c. Swallow (this will probably put air into your stomach and you will lose the air that's already trapped, so you will have to start over again).

    d. Pause and take some deep breaths. This is distracting if you are involved in a conversation, but you may not have any choice.

    e. Keep on talking. Sometimes the act of speaking (and therefore injecting air) will clear the bubble.

    f. Time! Although I still have the problem occasionally, the occurrences are not as frequent as time goes by. I'm not sure if this gradual control is because of conditioning or if the mind suppresses it subconsciously. The good news is that there is hope.

18. Establish set times for your practice. Self discipline is very important.

19. Exaggerate your mouth movement. You must be articulate!

20. Try to always practice with a mirror. Watch your mouth movement and check that you are not creating unusual or unnecessary expressions and movements.

21. Don't try to talk too fast. Think of speaking in a very slow, relaxed, deep voice. Speed and higher pitches will come with time. For now it's easier to speak slowly and in a deep monotone voice.

22. Never be satisfied with poor articulation. Repeat words that were not understandable. One of the most frustrating things for anyone is for someone to pretend that they understood you when they didn't.

23. Don't create a comfort zone that you stay within. Benefits are obtained by pushing beyond yesterday's limits.

24. Practice with a tape recorder. Not only is it important that you monitor your exercises by playing back the tapes, it's also nice to be able to play back some early tapes when you start feeling discouraged.

CHAPTER 4

HOW TO SPEAK

You have not lost your ability to speak. The laryngectomy that was performed on you merely removed the vocal cords that helped produce sound, and it eliminated the air passage between your lungs and mouth. You can still speak by forcing air through the esophagus to create sound, and that sound can still be converted into speech with your tongue, lips, teeth and gums. The only thing that's required is an air source to produce The Sound.

The Sound is created by injecting or inhaling air into the esophagus and trapping it until it's expelled. When the air is expelled it creates a vibration in the esophagus that results in a sound much like a burp or belch. In fact some people refer to esophageal speech as a controlled belch. Unlike a belch however, this sound does not come from the stomach if the air injection is done correctly. Many people have the misconception that esophageal speech is the result of swallowing air into the stomach and then forcing it out by constricting the muscles. A correct air injection only travels about 2 to 3 inches into the esophagus before it's trapped and controlled. You can achieve some speech by swallowing air into the stomach but it's very limited.

The ability to inject air into the esophagus on demand and control it is the basis of esophageal speech. Another way of forcing air into the esophagus is the consonant injection method which is described in Exercise 2 of this book. But, in order to become truly proficient at esophageal speech you must learn to rapidly inject air on demand, trap that air before it travels into the stomach, and control the rate of expulsion in order to speak.

There are many variations and descriptions of how to correctly inject air. The following description has been beneficial to numerous laryngectomees and I offer it with the hope that it may help you achieve The Sound.

Description of an air injection from "Self Help For The Laryngectomee" by Edmund Lauder:

"Imagine your mouth to be an empty paper bag -- you know that when you close the mouth of the bag you trap a good deal of the air in it. So it is with your mouth and the trapped air may eventually become the source of the sound. The idea is to physically move that "ball" of air which is trapped in your mouth to the back of your throat so that the air will enter and expand your esophagus and hopefully return in the form of that belch-like sound. Open your mouth (as if you were saying "ah"), then close it and compress your lips, compress your flattened tongue against the roof of your mouth and swallow the "ball" of air. As soon as you have done this, quickly open your mouth, pull in your stomach and attempt to say "PAH." Do this several times; if no sound is produced with "PAH" try doing the same thing and say "TAH" then "KAH".

In short, follow this pattern of actions:

1. Open the mouth.

2. Close the mouth, press the flattened tongue to the roof of your mouth and SWALLOW the "ball" of air all in one motion.

3. Quickly open the mouth, pull in your stomach and say "PAH" or "TAH" or "KAH."

If at all possible have an esophageal speaker show you how to do this. Your speech therapist may know someone that will give you a demonstration. If not, contact the local cancer society and see if they have any volunteers. Another possibility may be through a local Lost Cord Club. If all of those efforts fail or are unsuccessful, I offer the following description of how to make The Sound.

THE SOUND

I needed to express the process of injecting air a little differently to myself in order to more completely understand it and visualize what was occurring. Feelings are difficult to describe at best and what seems perfectly clear to you may create a different visual image to someone else. I had a hard time visualizing a "ball" of air moving from my mouth back into my throat. In your case that description may be perfectly obvious, the description below may seem better, or you may come up with something completely different.

Your primary objective at this point is to create a sound at will. However, you want that sound to originate high up in the esophagus instead of down in the stomach. This is accomplished by injecting air into the upper part of the esophagus and trapping it until it's expelled. I could not relate to descriptions of this action that refer to swallowing air or pushing a ball of air back with your tongue. I feel that a better description for me is to suck the air into your throat.

The simple act of just opening your mouth allows more than enough air to enter the oral cavity for speaking. The only action required on your part is to move that air back into the esophagus. The description that follows is not technical and it may sound crude. However, it is an explanation of something that everyone has done and I think it is the simplest way to force air into the esophagus.

    a. Close your mouth.

    b. Slightly puff your cheeks by filling them with air

    c. Close your eyes.

    d. Imagine that you have a bad cold and that your nose is plugged up. You have tried to blow your nose and nothing comes out, but you can feel the pressure of the mucus.

    e. Suck that mucus down into your throat so that you can spit it out.

This action of trying to suck imaginary mucus back into your throat will force (inject) air into your esophagus. You catch (trap) that air the same way you would catch the mucus before it reaches the stomach. *Let me make this as simple as I can! Imagine that you have snot in your nose. Now suck that snot into your throat and spit it out. The act of sucking that imaginary snot into your throat will force air into your esophagus.*

Now lets try to make a sound using the method above:

    a. Open your mouth to allow air in and then close it.

    b. Slightly puff your cheeks.

    c. Now with your mouth closed make a sucking motion.

    d. You should feel a soft thump at the back of your throat as the air is forced back and trapped. Concentrate on what you feel and hear.

    e. Concentrate on what's happening! Can you feel and hear a thump sound as the air is trapped? Try to exaggerate the sound of the thump until you can make the sound on demand. *Note: Once you have mastered the ability to create The Sound don't continue making loud thumping sounds.*

    f. Open your mouth wide and try to say "ah" (belch). Continue to do this until you can create a belch sound. Keep practicing until you can drag the sound out as in "ahhhhh."

Continue to practice making air injections and creating a belch sound until you can do it on demand. If my method does not seem to be working for you, try to create your own method by practicing different ways of belching. But remember, don't swallow air into your stomach on purpose. The sounds you create by that method are limited and hard to do on demand.

The rest of this manual consists of a series of exercises designed to assist you in converting The Sound into speech. The words and phrases are not random selections. They are arranged in an order that I found to be beneficial when I was learning to speak. As you discover which sounds and words are easiest for you to say you may want to rearrange them to fit your needs. Creating your own list of words also helps relieve some of the boring monotony of practice.

As you go through the exercises say each word at least three times before you go to the next word. Do not move on to the next exercise until you can say at least half of the words clearly. It would certainly be better if you could master all of the words before you continued, but some words are more difficult than others. I had a lot of problems with hard (long) vowel sounds and words that began with the letters "R" and "L". These may be easy for you, but then you may have trouble with another sound that was easy for me. One sound that we all have trouble with though is the "H" sound. The "H" will almost always be silent so don't try to say single words that start with "H". Most words beginning with "H" can be understood however if they are used in a sentence. For example "arry ad to get a aircut" can be understood quite easily.

There are no shortcuts. Do each lesson over and over until you have mastered every word and phrase. In order to progress you must increase the degree of difficulty as you move ahead. Only you know what is easy and what is difficult. Be proud of what you accomplish but never be satisfied with anything less than your goal.

CUPCAKE

~Jack Henslee

She approached with hesitation and uncertainty.
Still attractive at 73, despite the ravish of cancer
That had unmercifully destroyed her speech.
Her eyes reflected the fear and despair
Born from the pain of silence, darkened by sadness,
Quietly pleading for encouragement and hope.
Like most survivors she had many fears,
But most of all she wanted to talk.

Pen and paper were kept in hand, a substitute for speech.
In her purse, an electric device that simulated voice,
A lingering source of embarrassment
That constantly reminded her of the loss.
She joined the others that had preceded her
As she silently moved from the solitary darkness.
The long journey to self esteem had begun,
But most of all she wanted to talk.

The assault on silence began
With that mechanical voice she so despised.
Alien sounds tumbled precariously from her mouth,
Until the words started to slowly flow,
But the loneliness of silence had bred a deep depression.
With trembling lips and tear filled eyes
This newly acquired voice declared,
"I can speak, but most of all I want to talk."

Her lips drew taut, with a quivering tremble,
As her chosen quest was explained step by step.
The discipline to succeed, and the disappointments
That rage in dark fury were examined.
Her jaw drooped slightly from the weight of doubt,
But her eyes darkened with determination when she declared,
"I can do it, I know I can,
Because most of all I want to talk."

The quest began with a search for sound,
A simple Ah would be music, a word a symphony.
Scotch was repeatedly whispered until finally spoken,

Next came "Cup Cake", two words strung together
In a beautifully raspy voice, clearly understood.
She repeated, Cup Cake, Cup Cake, over and over,
Until her eyes filled with pride and joy.
Because most of all, now she could talk.

EXERCISE 1

This exercise consists of a list of single syllable words that start with sounds that are voiceless. In other words they can be said as a whisper without the use of vocal cords or esophageal speech. The intent of this exercise is not to teach you how to whisper words (speech is our goal) but to demonstrate that some limited communication already exists. While practicing these words and sounds pay close attention to the position of the tongue and the shape of the mouth. A good understanding of how to properly enunciate sounds will be useful in the later exercises. This exercise should not tire you so say each word at least three times, and spend at least fifteen minutes on it.

Remember: A journey of a thousand miles begins with one step.

TAP TACK TOP TIP TOOK TICK TAPE TAT

PIP PEEK PAP POT POP PUSH PICK PACK

CUP CAT COOK CAKE CHURCH COP CHASE

SCOTCH STEAK STEP SCRATCH SKATE SKIP

Did you concentrate on the tongue position and shape of the mouth? If you can whisper all of these words and you have a good feeling for how the tongue, in relationship to the mouth and teeth, produced these sounds, go to the next exercise.

EXERCISE 2

This exercise is a list of single syllable words or sounds to be spoken, not whispered. It is assumed that you have learned how to properly inject air and create the sound on demand. If you can't produce the sound yet, follow the instructions below for the consonant injection method. Try each word three times. Mark the ones that you have difficulty with and come back to them later.

TAP TIP TAKE TAPE TAT

SCOTCH STEAK STICK SCRATCH SPEAK

PIP PAP POP PUSH PACK PICK

CUP CAKE CHURCH CHEST CHOKE

This may seem like a short exercise but these are your first words with your new voice. Do not proceed to the next exercise until you can say at least half of these words clearly. Can you understand yourself on the tape recorder? Have someone listen to you. Can they understand you?

Consonant injection: If you have not learned how to make a correct air injection, and if you have put in at least two weeks or twenty hours of effort to learn, then try this method of speaking. This is only a temporary solution that will allow you to communicate in a limited capacity. You will be limited to words that start with certain consonants and short phrases that begin with certain consonants. In order to progress to connected conversational speech you will eventually have to learn to inject air on demand. However, I believe that at this point some limited speech is better than nothing, and although it is not my recommended choice of methods, it is the way that I learned.

a. Close your mouth and puff out your cheeks a little bit.

b. With your mouth closed, place your tongue at the roof of your mouth and behind your upper teeth.

c. Rapidly (with your mouth closed) make five or six "T" sounds (tuh, tuh, tuh, tuh, tuh), you should feel the air being forced into your esophagus.

d. Now, (by using the air you forced into your esophagus) say one of the "T" words above. This is done by using the air you pumped into your esophagus, to create a sound (belch or burp) when it's forced out. That sound is converted into speech with your tongue, teeth, and lips (Remember Exercise 1). You speak the same way as before, but with a different source of air for the sound.

e. Practice the rest of the words. Use the sounds of the consonants P, S, C and T to pump air into the esophagus.

Note: Another way to get a good feel of the air being pumped back into the esophagus is to try saying the letter "K" with your mouth closed. You may also want to slightly flex or tense your stomach muscles when you force the air out. In my case I am not aware of any involvement from my stomach and therefore I don't feel that it is necessary. This method has been beneficial to others however and you should try anything that may help you.

Practice these words until you feel comfortable with them. Make a list of the ones that seem easy and another list of the ones that you have trouble with. Use the easy ones to warm up with before an exercise. Go back to the hard ones after you have progressed a little farther. Try to analyze why some are easy and others are hard.

EXERCISE 3

This exercise is a list of single syllable words that begin with a consonant and have a soft (short) vowel sound. These consonants represent sounds that I feel are the easiest to make. You will notice that most of these are "voiceless" words that create some air resistance inside the mouth when producing the sound of the consonant.

These words are also ideal for consonant injection because the act of speaking them helps pump air into the esophagus. Later on you will see that by using a lot of words with these sounds you can reduce the number of air injections required to speak.

This is where the work begins. Do not skip this exercise! Do not continue until you can say at least half of these words! Practice, practice, and then practice some more. This is the beginning and you may be one of the lucky ones who are successful after a couple of days, or you may be like me and take a few weeks. Don't give up! You can do it!

TAH   TAP   TAT   TALK   TICK

TOT   TIE   TACK   TAB   TED

PAH   PAT   PACK   POT   PUCK

PASS   PILL   PAN   PIN   PIT

CAP   CAT   COT   CAN   COW

CAR   CHOW   CHUCK   CHEW   CHEST

SAP   STAB   SAT   STEW   SACK

SIT   SCAT   SPIT   SCAN   SEND

EXERCISE 4

These are more single syllable words with soft vowel sounds. The consonant sounds are a little harder than the ones in exercise 3, but if you can do exercise 3 then you can do this.

GAP GAS GOT GOOD GOD

BAP BASS BACK BAT BALL

BILL BEST BATCH BOX BED

DAN DOG DOT DO DEAD

SUCK SPEND SHIN SPOT SPIN

FAT FALL STALL FILL SKILL

FAN SKIN FIT KIT BUS

MAN VAN MUST STICK MAKE

STILL KICK MUD TICK DOWN

CHILL CHIN CALL SHOT KILL

TEST PICK KIN BIT PILL

Before you go on to exercise 5 make a list of 40 words from exercises 3 and 4 and practice them. Start with an easy word and then a hard word. In most cases you will find that if you say an easy word first, then the hard word is easier to say if you say it immediately after the easy word.

You may also discover that if you repeat the same word immediately that it sounds better the second time. The reason that the second word seems easier is because the first word acts as the pump to inject air into the esophagus. This natural action will be very useful when you start speaking in short phrases.

EXERCISE 5

These words all start with consonants just like in the first 4 exercises, but these words either have a hard vowel sound or a double vowel sound. I had a lot of trouble with these types of sounds because when you produce a vowel sound there is very little air resistance inside the mouth. Since there was little or no resistance, most of the air I injected would escape before I could finish the word. Take your time with this exercise. After you have mastered this the rest should be easy!

TIME   TREAT   TAKE   TAME   TOW

SPEECH   SLIT   SLOW   SAME   SHOW

PLAY   PEAT   PAY   PLAN   PRAY

CLAY   CLAN   CLOCK   CLEAR   CROW

MAY   MUST   MY   MAKE   MOW

BLANK   BAKE   BEAT   BANK   BOW

SAY   SNAKE   CHEAT   NEAT   SNOW

RAY   RAKE   RIGHT   RICKY   ROW

GRAY   GAME   GRAB   GRIT   GROW

STAY   FLAME   PLEAT   QUIT   FLOW

Before you go on to the next exercise practice the alphabet. This will give you an idea of which sounds are still hard. Also try counting up to 100. Counting will help you improve your speed plus it introduces you to multiple syllables.

EXERCISE 6

This exercise is simply to test your articulation. Say these words to a monitor (listener) and/or into your recorder. Can you tell the difference between these sound-alike words?

CAME / FAME   SOW / GLOW   NAME / SHAME   SLIGHT / LIKE

SLAB / CRAB   SPEND / MEND   TALL / MALL   SEND / BEND

CLOT / SLOT   BLAB / SCAB   TRAIL / SNAIL   RING / FLING

TIGHT / FLIGHT   KING / SPRING   BRIGHT / FIGHT   SAIL / FAIL

BRING / STRING   FRANK / BANK   FLAME / BLAME   SIT / BIT

BRAND / SAND   DOCK / KNOCK   CLICK / BRICK   STOP / SHOP

SHAKE / FAKE   SEAT / NEAT   EACH / REACH   REAR / FEAR

EXERCISE 7

This exercise consists of 2 syllable words. You should be able to produce a consonant or vowel sound on demand by this time, and your articulation should be fairly good (about 75% of what you say should be understandable). If you have not progressed to this level go back and practice some more. It is not necessary that you can say all of the words in the preceding exercises, but the ones that you can say should be understandable. This exercise will help you extend your sound production per air injection, and that will help you produce more words per injection. You may even find that some of these words are actually easier than some of the single syllable words.

At first you may need to pause after the first syllable (tur / key, bas / ket etc). Don't worry about it. You will be able to smooth the words out into a single sound after some practice.

CAREFUL   BROTHER   GARDEN   MOTIVE   STOMA

COVER   BREAKFAST   GRAVY   MASTERPIECE   SKINNY

COMING   BASKET   GUPPIES   MULTITUDE   SUBMERGE

COFFEE   BABY   GARLIC   MORNING   SPOKEN

CONTAIN   BUTTER   GENTLE   MOVING   SUBMARINE

CHICKEN   BACON   GRAPEFRUIT   MUSTARD   SPINACH

CABBAGE   PEPPER   TABLE   MONOTONE   ALMOST

CARROTS   PERHAPS   TURKEY   FOOLPROOF   ALWAYS

CANDY   PEOPLE   BEFORE   FATHER   APPLE

PROMOTION   BETWEEN   FALSEHOOD   ACHIEVE   LUCKY

DOZEN   DRAGSTER   BANDAGE   FIGURE   ADDRESS

EXERCISE 8

This exercise is really a continuation of exercise 7 except that instead of a single 2 syllable word, it consists of 2 single syllable words that form a phrase. If you have to pause between words at first it's OK. But before you continue you should be able to say each phrase without a noticeable pause, and with only one air injection.

GOOD NIGHT   CALL ME   SHAKE HANDS   SIT DOWN

CHEER UP   NICE DAY   PAY DAY   COME IN

DON'T GO   I KNOW   RIGHT NOW   GET OUT

PLEASE STAY   GOOD BYE   GOOD MORNING   BE QUIET

GOOD SHOT   THANK YOU   COME HERE   TELL ME

NO THANKS   STAND UP   SOME DAY   SPEAK UP

KEEP IT   BREAK TIME   PLAY BALL   DO IT

NOON TIME   BED TIME   RIGHT NOW   COME BACK

VERY GOOD   PARDON ME   TRY AGAIN   THAT'S NICE

THAT'S BAD   GOOD JOB   WHY NOT   CALL ME

LET'S EAT   LET'S GO   CATCH HIM   STOP THAT

NOW WHAT   THAT'S GOOD   TALK SLOW   GOOD JOB

Before you move on to the next exercise take some time and make a list of additional phrases from the words that you have learned. In the early stages of developing your new voice a strong vocabulary of short phrases is very beneficial. Practice phrases that you would normally use until they become automatic. As you become proficient add more words to create sentences like "No thanks, keep it," or "Try again someday."

EXERCISE 9

This exercise is composed of short phrases or statements that have 3 or more syllables. Practice these until you can say each phrase and then practice until you can say them with only one air injection.

THANK THE MAN   THANK YOU SIR   CATCH THE BALL

HOW ARE YOU   PASS THE SALT   STOP THE CAR

TIME TO TALK   TIME TO EAT   TAKE YOUR TIME

LISTEN TO THIS   PET THE CAT   FEED THE DOG

TIME FOR BED   GET UP NOW   LET'S GO OUT

COMB YOUR HAIR   ARE YOU COLD   I AM FINE

SEE YOU SOON   TIME TO SHOUT   TIME TO PRAY

THEY ARE GOOD   ARE THEY GOOD   CAN YOU COUNT

YOU CAN COUNT   ARE YOU FINE   YOU ARE FINE

CAN YOU STAND   YOU CAN STAND   THIS IS GOOD

KEEP IT SIMPLE   CHARLIE SHOT SKIP   SKIP SHOT CHARLIE

LET'S EAT NOW   THIS IS EASY   TAKE IT SLOW

DO IT NOW   PIECE OF CAKE   TIME FOR DINNER

POLISH YOUR SHOES   USE BLACK POLISH   TAKE IT EASY

LISTEN TO ME   FANTASTIC JOB   TAKE A BREAK

EXERCISE 10

This is a list of much longer statements. Take a pause where you see slash marks (/), and an air injection if you need one. As you get stronger you will be able to move the slashes mark farther and farther to the right until you can say the entire statement with only one air injection.   Remember what I said earlier about certain consonant sounds automatically pumping air into the esophagus? This is where you find out how well it really works.

TAKE TIME / TO TALK.

LET'S GO / OUT FOR DINNER.

TAKE OUT / THE GARBAGE.

DON'T GO / IT'S TOO EARLY.

DO YOU / PLAY GOLF?

WOULD YOU / LIKE TO LEARN?

DID YOU / SLEEP WELL?

I'M GOING / TO THE STORE.

DID YOU BAKE / A CAKE TODAY?

HOW MUCH / DO I / OWE YOU?

HOW MUCH / DOES IT COST?

WHERE ARE / MY KEYS?

WHERE IS / THE CAR?

I NEED / TO TALK / TO YOU.

WHERE / ARE YOU GOING?

LETS GO OUT / FOR DINNER.

DON'T FORGET / THE TIP.

WOULD YOU LIKE / A DRINK?

IT'S COLD / OUTSIDE.

WHEN IS / MY APPOINTMENT?

CAN YOU / UNDERSTAND ME?

THAT WAS / VERY GOOD.

TO SPEAK WELL / TAKES A LOT / OF TIME. / LET'S GET / TO WORK.

EXERCISE 11

Practice these phrases until you can say them with one air injection.

A MAN SHOWS WHAT HE IS
        BY WHAT HE DOES
                WITH WHAT HE HAS.

    A SHIP IN A HARBOR IS SAFE,
        BUT THAT'S NOT WHAT SHIPS ARE BUILT FOR.

       THE RACE IS NOT ALWAYS TO THE SWIFT,
BUT TO THOSE WHO KEEP ON RUNNING.

       STRIVING FOR SUCCESS WITHOUT HARD WORK
IS LIKE TRYING TO HARVEST WHERE YOU HAVEN'T PLANTED .

     MINDS ARE LIKE PARACHUTES;
      THEY ONLY WORK WHEN THEY'RE OPEN.

LIFE IS A ROAD OF THORNS,
    WITH A ROSE EVERY FEW HUNDRED MILES.

      TODAYS SUCCESS WAS YESTERDAYS LIMIT.

TOMORROW'S ACHIEVEMENTS HAVE NO LIMIT.

Continue to practice these phrases until you can say the entire phrase with only one air injection. When you can do that you are ready for the final chapter.

Chapter 5

CONVERSATIONAL SPEECH

I thought that this would be the easy part. After all I could inject air on demand, I could say almost any word I wanted, or at least substitute it with another word, and I could do 9 to 12 syllables per injection. I was very wrong!

All of the great things that I had accomplished required a lot of concentration and a conscious effort to inject air, produce a sound, and articulate words. In a way I had trained myself to do some tricks. Nothing was natural. I had to think about what I wanted to say, think about injecting air, think about how to position and move my mouth, and control my breathing all at the same time.

It simply was not possible to converse at any length until some of these actions became subconscious responses. Even now my subconscious will sometimes fail me and I have a breakdown in coordinating all of the necessary actions. When this happens I have to slow everything down to regain control and establish a rhythm. Once you can create sound at will and easily speak short phrases, then rhythm becomes the main key to learning how to converse. The only advice I can give for this phase is to disassociate the breathing from the speaking and practice, practice and then practice some more.

The entire process of esophageal speech is simply training, exercising, and conditioning the esophagus to inject and control air within a small area of the esophagus. It takes a lot of hard work to build up the required strength, and your progress can only be maintained by speaking a lot through normal conversation or practice sessions. Use it or lose it!

You should now be at a point where you can say any word you desire and you can probably speak a minimum of seven to nine syllables per air injection. You must now learn how to combine all of those words, syllables, and phrases that you worked so hard to master into connected conversational speech.

One of the best exercises I've found for practicing this is to read children's poetry out loud. There is something about the rhythm and simple phrasing that seems to help in extending speech. Even today I sometimes have a hard time reading anything else out loud. It appears that even though my speech seems to be natural, a lot of subconscious concentration still takes place. It's very difficult to read and speak at the same time while trying to maintain your rhythm of breathing, injecting air, and understanding what your reading.

Go to the library and find some light reading material (preferably children's poetry) and read it out loud. Try to find poems that are about 80 to 120 words long. Record your readings and then count how many words per minute you can read. When you can speak at a rate of 60 words per minute you are on your way. When you have mastered the easy poems, then you can move on to more lengthy and complex readings, like the Sounds of Silence, or Cupcake. Once you can speak at a sustained rate of 80 or more words per minute you are considered to be a proficient esophageal speaker. There may still be some frustrating times. You have made a lot of progress and put in a lot of hard work to get this far. Just by using your new voice every day you will continue to improve. The progress may seem slow and unnoticeable at this point but it is occurring. How much farther you want to go is up to you !

About the Author

Jack Henslee is a 3 time neck cancer survivor (1979, 1988, & 1995) and a stage 3 lung cancer survivor in 2013.

Founded the Look Who's Talking Lost Chord Club in Stockton CA. (1989)

Officer and Board Member of the California Association of Laryngectomees since 1992 and is the current Chairman of the Board.

Joined the International Association of Laryngectomees in1991 and has served as board member, Vice President, Treasurer, and Executive Director.

Created the Voices Restored Project in 2008 which has donated over 100 speech aids, supplies, and some speech training to Costa Rica, Peru, and the Philippines.

Produced the award winning documentary "Voices Restored – Costa Rica" which took a first place award at the 2010 Costa Rica International Film Festival.

Member and contributing writer and editor for the WebWhispers Nu-Voice Club (www.webwhispers.org)

www.ingramcontent.com/pod-product-compliance
Lightning Source LLC
Chambersburg PA
CBHW081359170526
45166CB00010B/3140